Natural DIY Homemade Hand Sanitizer and Wipes
Recipes with natural essential oils for Healthy
Living and Germ Free Home

Introduction

The best and most traditional way to get your hands clean is washing them with soap and water. But there are situations when sink is not available for the washing hand sanitizer is an excellent and ideal solution to this dilemma and it's so simple to make it at home. Making hand sanitizer at home is also an excellent project for both children and adults to participate also it is much more economical and the fact that you get a quality product that keeps you and your family safe from germs and you can even give it out as gift items

Frequent washing of the hands and the using alcohol-based hand sanitizer are regarded as the best ways to prevent infection. Hand hygiene is popular recognized as one of the most important ways in the prevention of infection. Health care system states that the major cause of death and disability are infections. Proper hand hygiene is the best way to prevent the spread of pathogens and reduction in infections The World Health Organization and U.S. Center for Disease Control provided guidelines for proper hand hygiene and carry out studies and survey to measure the effectiveness of these hand sanitizers The surveys showed that the fastest and most effective way to eliminate germs and reduce infections is with hand sanitizers.as it is simple, effective, and well tolerated.

Effective Hand Washing

Follow these guidelines while washing your hands

* Place your hands under a clean, running water (warm or cold), to wet them, then smear soap (liquid or solid) on your hands.
* Rub the hands together with the soap to lather it Lather the backs of your hands, between your fingers, and under your nails.
* Scrub your hands for a minimum of 20 seconds. Proceed to rinse your hands well under clean, running water.
* using a clean towel, disposable paper towel or air-dry to dry your hands.

Though washing of hand with soap where possible is still better, but in situations where soap and water is not available hand, sanitizer is handy.

Hand sanitizer have both active and inactive ingredients. Inactive ingredients contain water, a thickening agent like polyacrylic acid that gives gel hand sanitizers its structure sometimes fragrance or color are added to the sanitizer. For the active Ingredients approved by the Food and Drug Administration and Centers Disease Control and Prevention are alcohol and providine-iodine. Providine-iodine is not so popular but the alcohol formulations have been widely adopted and approved also by World Health Organization.

We have different forms of hand sanitizer, they includes gels, foams, liquids and wipes. Individuals may prefer one form to the other. Different forms of hand sanitizers are shown in Table below

Type	. Description	Comments
Liquid	Water-like sanitizer that	Rapid dispersal across surfaces,

	can be put in to a spray bottle	the concern is that it might be dripping and also can cause wetness of the surface
Gel	Jelly-like colloid dispersed in a semisolid form	Commonly used, well tolerated, can leave "stickiness" on the hands
Foam	A mass of small bubbles formed from the infusion of air in to solution	Created during manual activation of a dispenser or air pressurized canister
Wipe	Small cloth or fabric soaked in antimicrobial solution	Effective at removing dirt and foreign material from the hands

1

Table 1. Hand Sanitizer Forms.

Take Note

Ensure that the bottles for the sanitizer are well labelled and kept out of the reach of toddlers, to avoid accidental ingestion

Get hand gloves while preparing it to avoid any form of contamination although if alcohol is being used it can effectively kills the germs but for those with sensitive skin to protect your hand mixing the ingredients

Store hand sanitizers in a cool dry place.

Liquid Hand Sanitizer Recipes

Home Made Gel Hand Sanitizer Recipes

There are several options for making an all-natural homemade hand sanitizer gel. However, we are going to be making one that is lightweight and easy to dry gel. And all natural ones also

Clear Water Base Gel:

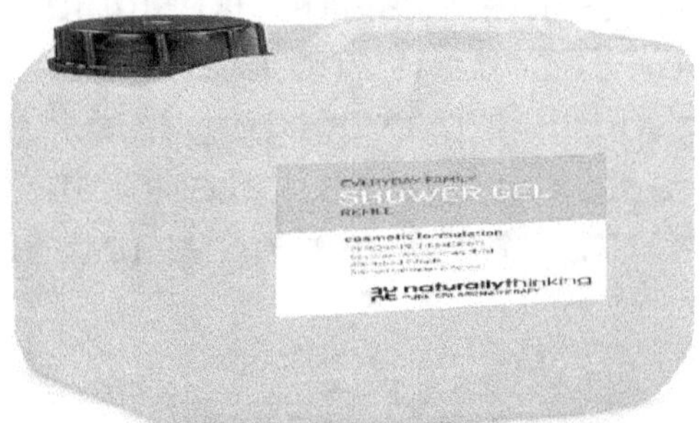

Water base gel are non-greasy light, cooling, moisturizing and has a soothing quality. It is oil free and hydrating.

Glycerin

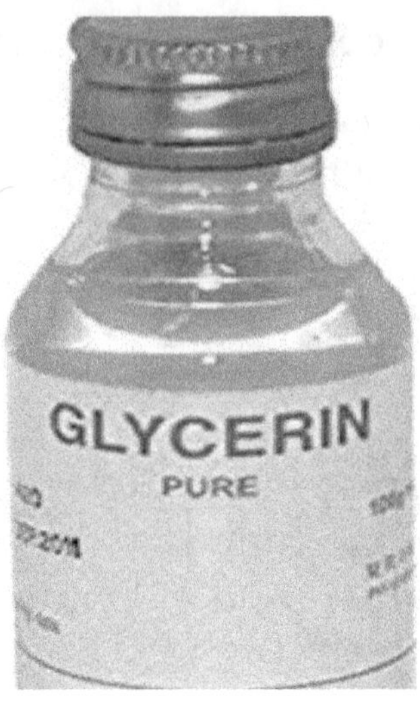

Glycerin, also known as glycerol or glycerin, is usually a colorless, odorless, syrup like liquid with a sweet flavor. It softens and keeps the skin supple, therefore will prevent the dryness that the alcohol content of the sanitizer might cause. It is also anti-bacterial and great for sensitive skins

Propylene Glycol

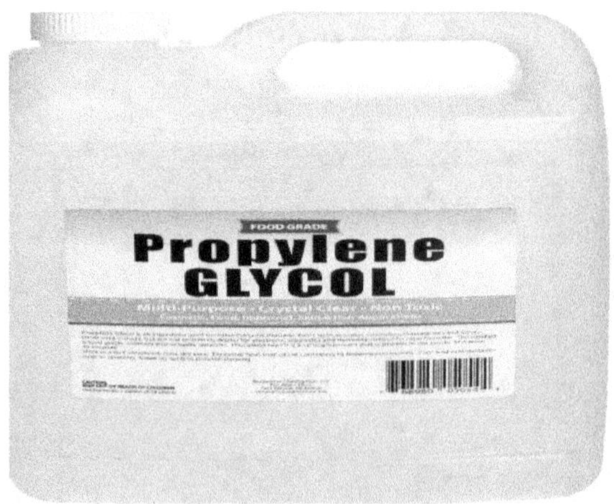

Propylene glycol is an organic compound, the chemical formula is CH3CH(OH)CH2OH. It is a thick and colorless liquid, and is odorless but has a light sweet taste

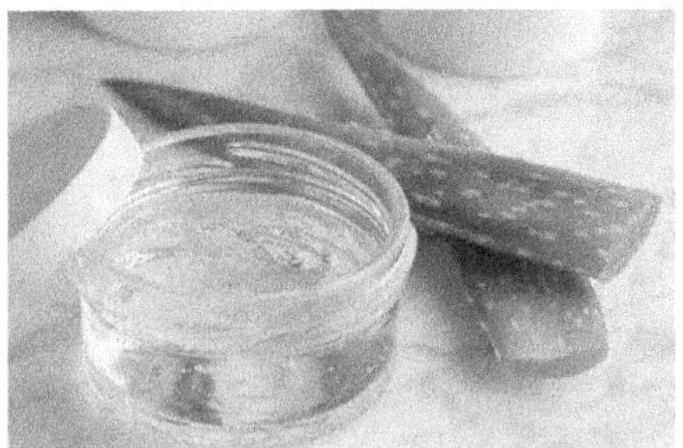

Aloe Vera gel is extracted from the aloe Vera leaves. It can be taken orally in liquid or capsule form. It is good for various kinds of skin treatments including burns and other various skin conditions. The Aloe Vera gel eases irritation, help with cold and acnes. It stops itching and inflammation

Isopropyl Alcohol

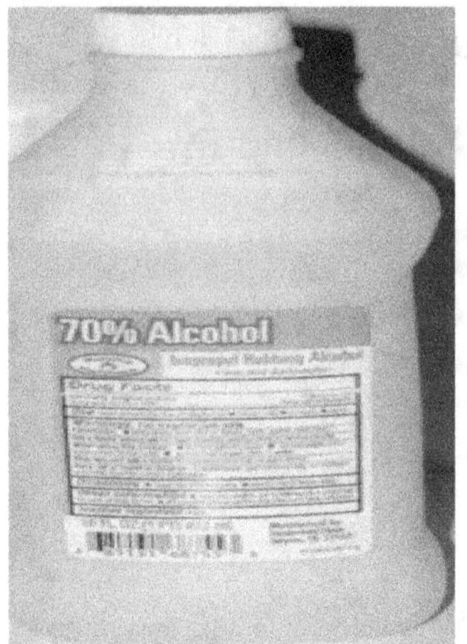

Isopropyl alcohol with 99% alcohol is the WHO recommended choice for making of hand sanitizer. It is colorless with a strong odor.

It is used in the manufacturing of many industrial and household products such as antiseptics, disinfectants, and detergents.

Tea Tree oil

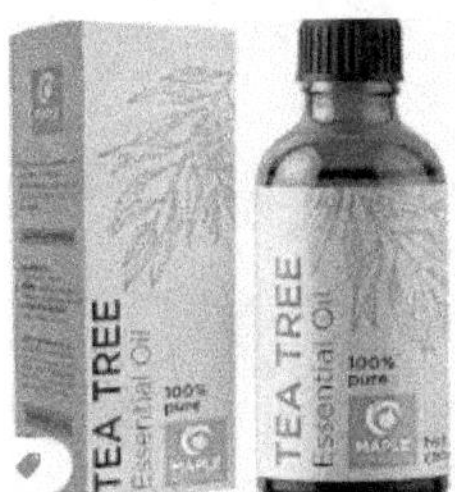

Tea tree oil is a great recommendation for hand sanitizer and disinfectants because of its anti-inflammatory and antimicrobial properties. It reduce redness, swelling, and inflammation. It could help to prevent, reduce, and fade acne scars, giving you a smooth, clear skin

Jojoba Oil

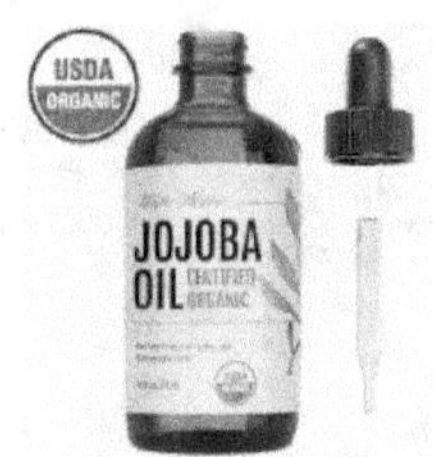

jojoba oil help to reduce chaffing and chapping, reduce redness caused by drying due to its anti-inflammatory properties, it keeps the skin calm and comfortable. The Vitamin E and B-complex vitamins found in the Jojoba oil help in skin repair and damage control

Tools you will need:

A clean bowl

A spatula or spoon,

 A funnel and a recycled liquid soap or hand sanitizer bottle if you do not have any, just get an empty spray bottle on hand

Quick Light easy to dry Hand Gel Sanitizer Recipe

45g of Water Base Gel

1g - Glycerin

1g - Propylene Glycol

1-5g - Aloe Vera Gel Extract

52.5g - Isopropyl Alcohol

0.5g – Essential Oil (Tea tree oil or jojoba oil)

- ❖ Combine the ingredients
- ❖ Stir vigorously with your spatula or spoon until all the ingredients are fully mixed together
- ❖ If you do not want to stir with your spatula, you can use your food processor to get a smooth mixture. Ensure to wash and rinse the food processor properly
- ❖ with your funnel pour the mixture into your bottle

The mixture can be kept for six months or more .store in a cool dry place, away from direct sunlight to get the longest shelf life possible.

You can put the mixture in smaller bottles that will be portable to carry in a purse, wallet, brief case or backpack for use on the go. Or give away as gift items

Nature made scented Hand Sanitizer

This natural gel hand sanitizer can done using the following ingredients

- ❖ 5 drops of tea tree oil
- ❖ 5 drops of lavender oil
- ❖ 3 drops of witch hazel
- ❖ 3 tbsp. of Aloe Vera Gel
- ❖ 1 tbsp. of Vitamin E oil (as emollient)

Directions

Combine all the ingredient in a bottle and check vigorously until an even mixture is obtain

Store and use

Alcohol-Based Hand Sanitizer with three ingredients

- ❖ Two third cup of rubbing alcohol (isopropyl alcohol)
- ❖ 1/3 cup of pure natural aloe Vera gel (for thickening)
- ❖ 7 to 10 drops of glycerin (or any essential oil of your choice preferably non-phototoxic oil like tea tree oil to avoid sunburn)
- ❖ Mixing bowl
- ❖ Spoon
- ❖ Funnel
- ❖ Recycled hand sanitizer

Direction

Combine the alcohol with aloe Vera gel in a bowl and mix it well if it is too thick add a little more alcohol and if it is too watery add a little more of the aloe Vera gel add the essential oil and mix to get a smooth mixture . Then transfer the mixture to your recycled hand sanitized bottle cap and store

Natural Awesome Anti-viral hand sanitizer
This awesome homemade hand sanitizer is all-natural and has anti –viral and anti-bacterial properties. It is a cocktail of essential oils. In addition, it is toxic free.

Ingredients

- ❖ A recycled spray bottle or hand sanitizer
- ❖ 7 drops of vitamin E oil (great for softening of hands)
- ❖ 2 tsp of witch hazel
- ❖ 2 tsp. of aloe Vera gel
- ❖ Optional 2 tsp of vodka (since we have witch hazel, which will do the same thing as the vodka).
- ❖ 6 drops lemon oil
- ❖ 6 drops orange oil
- ❖ 6 drops tea tree oil
- ❖ Boiled, cooled and filtered water

Directions

1. In the spray bottle which is about 2 ounce, combine all the oils (vitamin E witch hazel or vodka, orange, lemon tea tree.) cap the bottle and shake very well to get a uniform mix
2. Add the distilled water and shake for 15 seconds

If you have a label, sheet write hand sanitizer on it and stick it to the bottle or use a paper and a transparent, tape and stick it o on the bottle.
Use as needed

Homemade Hand Sanitizer Recipe from WHO

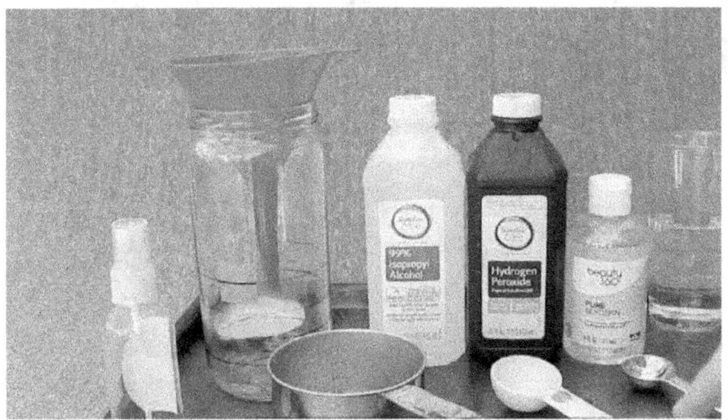

Ingredients

1 cup of Isopropyl alcohol 99%

1 Tsp. of hydrogen peroxide 3%

I tsp of glycerin

½ cup of Distilled water

 A recycled hand sanitizer bottle or a spray bottle.

Directions

 Combine all the ingredients in a glass jar, place the lid and shake gently to mix well

 Then pour in the spray bottle use as needed

Tips warnings and Precautions

Exercise precautions when handling essential oils they are in a raw form and are powerful plant extracts. If this is your first time of using them , carry out a patch test to check for any allergic reaction For a quick simple patch test add one drop of the oil you want to use (lavender, lemon or orange)to one tablespoon of olive oil. Rub a little of it on the inside of your elbow, cover with a bandage; leave it for a day to see if there is any negative or uncomfortable reaction.

Note that the lavender used the recipe is to reduce the dominating scent of the tea tree oil. If you do not like the scent of lavender, you can replace it with other antibacterial oil like Rosemary, sage, sandalwood, or peppermint

Bear in mind that essential oils are natural anti-inflammatory! However, for those with sensitive skin, you may want to stay away from lemon and orange oils because it can cause photosensitivity—meaning they make your skin more sensitive to sun exposure.

Better still you just want to buy off the shelf already pre-blended essential oil that is on the market which safe for kids also
Both vodka and witch hazel have natural anti-microbial properties (although alcohol is stronger and better at destroying germs), so either of them is ok.

Also dark bottles or amber ones are best for storing this hand sanitizer to help protect the essential oils from UV light (which can break them down),

This Do it yourself cleaning wipes recipes will make cleaning easy and save your some money. The following simple ingredients are required

Isopropyl Alcohol

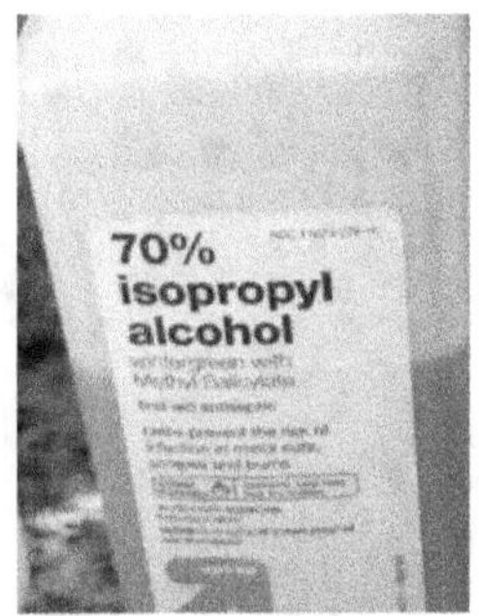

Thick Plain Paper Towel

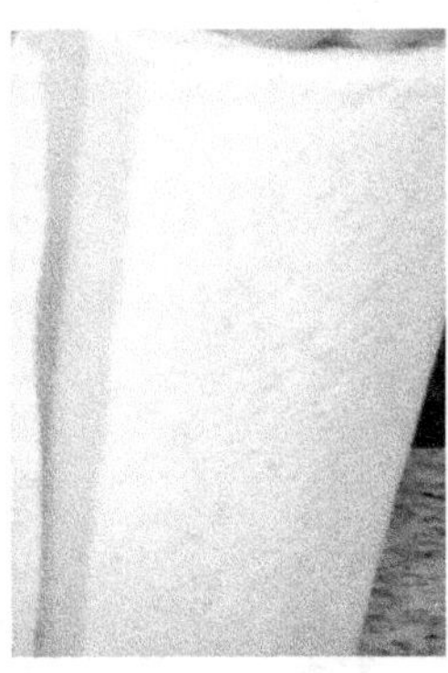

Dish washing Liquid

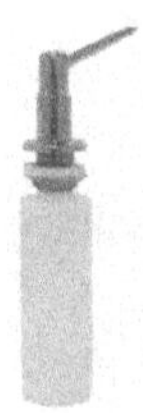

A container with a tight-fitting lid

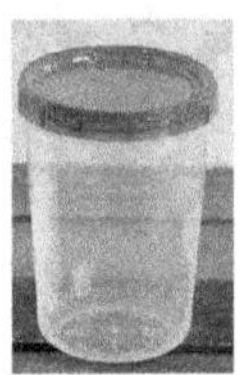

Distilled Water

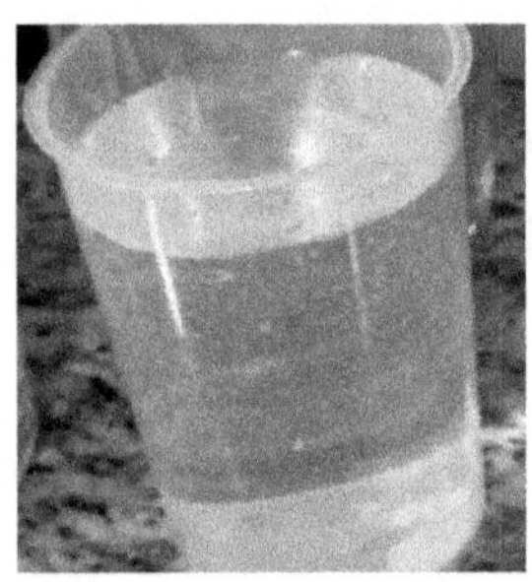

Baking Soda and lemon

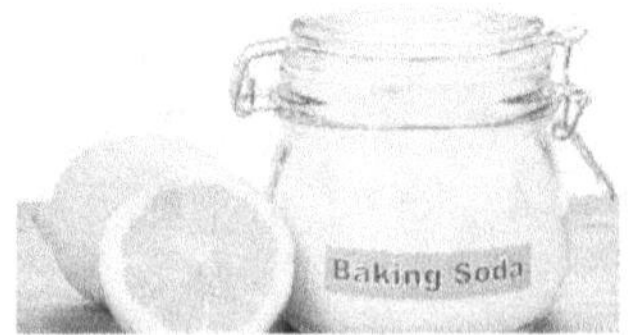

Distilled White Vinegar

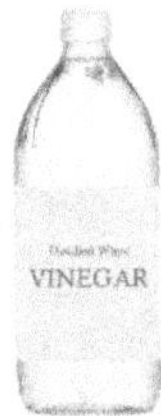

Lemon Oil

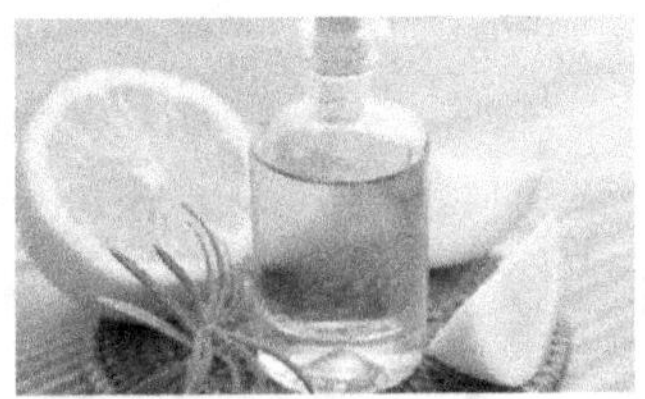

Lavender oil

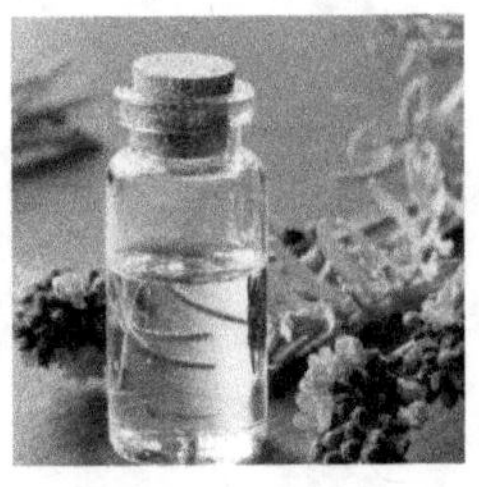

Tea Tree oil

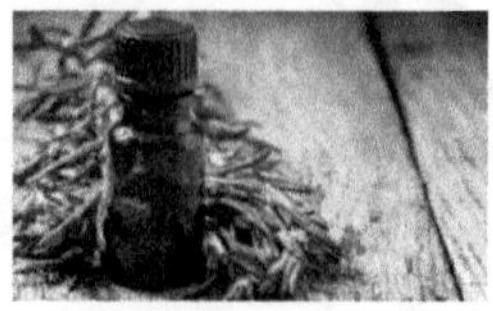

Wash cloth

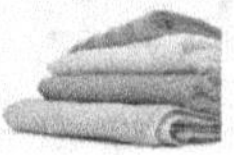

Glass Jar

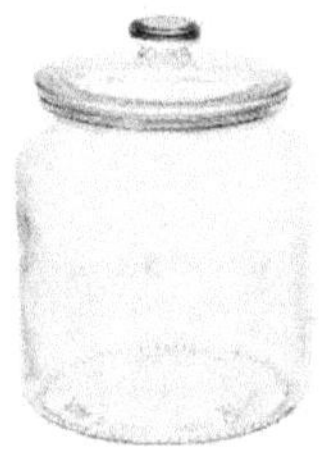

Spatula and Serrated Knife

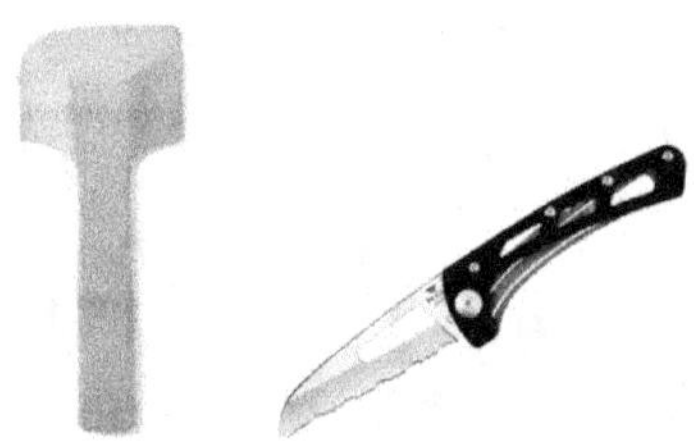

Reusable Homemade Cleaning Wipes

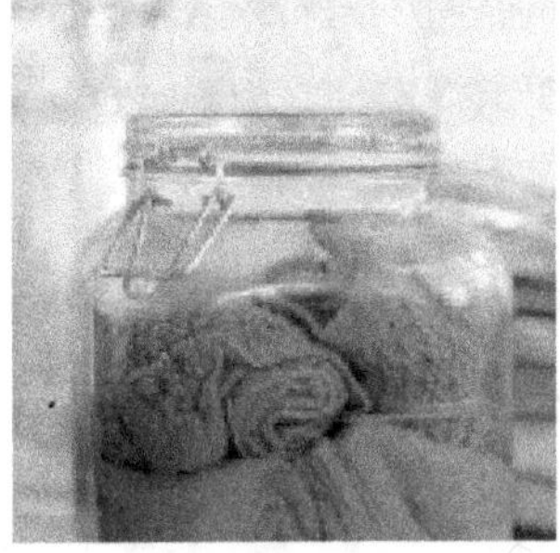

Ingredients
- ❖ One cup of distilled water
- ❖ One cup of distilled white vinegar
- ❖ 15 drops of Lemon oil
- ❖ 1 tablespoon of lemon juice
- ❖ 1 tablespoon of baking soda
- ❖ 15 drops of Lavender oil
- ❖ 2 drops of dish washing Liquid

Directions
- ❖ Fold the washcloths and place in the glass jar.
- ❖ Get a small bowl, Add the distilled water, Dish liquid wash ,white vinegar and the oils(lavender, Lemon)
- ❖ Mix the baking soda and lemon juice with a little distilled water in another container stir until evenly mixed
- ❖ Pour the two mixtures over the washcloths in a jar, use a spatula to press the washcloths down into the

liquid. Until the washcloths are wet, add
more vinegar or water as needed.
* Close the lid on the jar.
* Remove and use the washcloths for
instant wiping and cleaning of the floor
as needed if the washcloth get dirty
wash and repeat the process of soaking
in the prepared mixture the wipes
should be used within a week.

. Note that this wipe is not for granite, marble,
or other natural stone surfaces.

Alcohol Based Reusable Homemade

Cleaning Wipes

Ingredients
* 2 cups of distilled water
* 1/4 cup of Isopropyl Alcohol
* 2 drops of Dish washing Liquid
* 10 drops of Lavender oil
* 10 drops of Lemon oil

Directions
Combine all the ingredients in the jar. Put the lid
on and shake gently to get an even mixture

After the mixture is well combined, add your
cleaning cloths to the jar. The washcloth should be
wet

Replace the lid on the jar, and then turn the jar
upside-down for a while to ensure complete
absorption.

The wash cloth is ready for use

Disinfecting Bleach Wipes with plain Paper towel

Ingredients

- ❖ 2 tablespoons Bleach
- ❖ 2 1/2 cups of water
- ❖ A container with tight fitting lid
- ❖ Half roll of plain paper towel
- ❖ Serrated knife

Directions

Cut your paper towel into two using the serrated knife

Place the hall roll paper towel in the airtight container

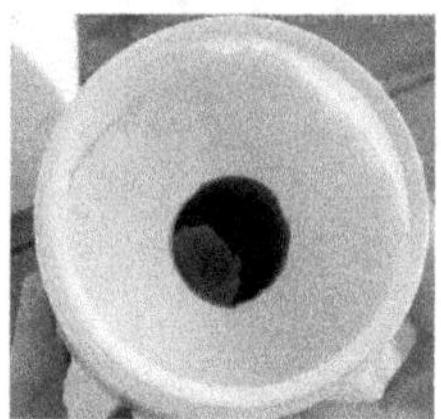

Mix the bleach and the water in a bowl and pour it over the paper towel until it is wet, allow it to sit for a while and then remove the cardboard in the center of the paper towel

You can take a paper towel from the middle so that it is taken from the center

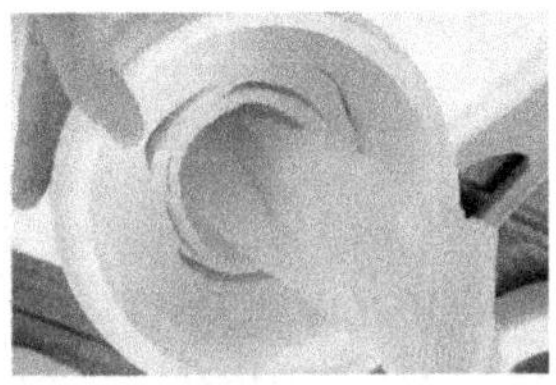

That is it

Disinfecting Wipes with plain Paper towel (Alcohol Based)

Ingredients

- ❖ 2 cups of distilled water
- ❖ 1/4 cup of Isopropyl Alcohol
- ❖ 2 drops of Dish washing Liquid
- ❖ 10 drops of Lavender oil
- ❖ A container with tight fitting lid
- ❖ Half roll of plain paper towel
- ❖ Serrated knife

Directions

Cut your paper towel into two using the serrated knife

Place the half roll paper towel in the airtight container

Get a small bowl, Add the distilled water, dishwashing liquid and the lavender oil mix well and pour over the paper towel.

Allow to sit for a while and then remove the cardboard in the center of the paper towel

You can take a paper towel from the middle so that it is taken from the center

Place the lid over it and use as needed

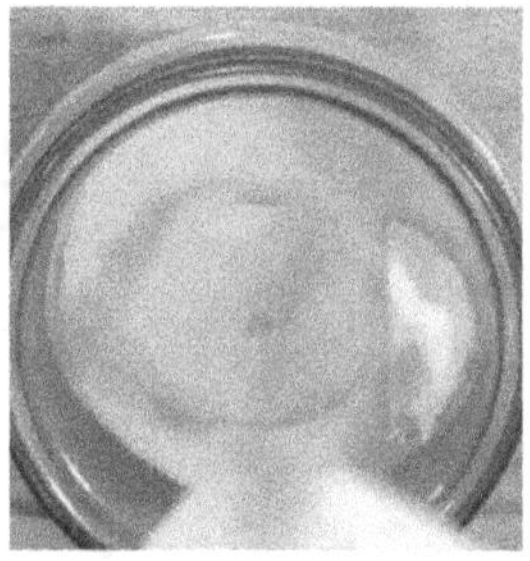

Home Made Make up Remover Wipes

Ingredients

* 3 cups of warm water
* 2 tsp. of coconut oil or olive oil
* 2 drops of tea tree oil
* 2 drops of baby wash or any of your favorite face wash (optional)
* A container with tight fitting lid
* Half roll of plain paper towel or cloths

Directions

Place the half roll paper towel in the airtight container

Get a small bowl, combine the warm water, the oils, mix well and pour over the paper towel.

Allow to sit for a while and then remove the cardboard in the center of the paper towel

Use as needed

DIY Homemade Natural Baby Wipes recipe

Ingredients

* 2 cups of distilled water
* 2 tsp. of aloe Vera gel
* 2 tsp. of liquid castile soap or mild baby wash liquid
* 2 tsp of alcohol free witch hazel

- ❖ A container with tight fitting lid
- ❖ Half roll of plain paper towel
- ❖ Half tsp. of fractionated coconut oil
- ❖ 15 drops tea tree oil
- ❖ 15 drops of lavender oil

Direction

Place the half roll paper towel in the airtight container

Get a small bowl, combine all the ingredients, mix well and pour over the paper towel. Until it is wet

Allow to sit for a while and then remove the cardboard in the center of the paper towel

Use as needed

This recipe is same if you are using reusable cloths

Anti-Fungal Baby Wipes Recipe

This is great for treating and prevent yeast infection rashes.

Ingredients

* One cup filtered water
* One tsp calendula oil
* 5 drops lavender oil
* 5 drops tea tree oil
* Half cup of aloe Vera gel
* Half roll of plain paper towel
* A container with tight fitting lid

Direction

Place the half roll paper towel in the airtight container

Get a small bowl, combine all the ingredients, mix well and pour over the paper towel. Until it is wet

Allow to sit for a while and then remove the cardboard in the center of the paper towel

Use as needed

Cocktail of Lavender and Tea Tree Oil Wipes for Rash Prevention

Ingredients

* 7 drops of olive oil

- ❖ 2 cups of filtered water
- ❖ -1 tsp baby wash
- ❖ Half roll of plain paper towel
- ❖ A container with tight fitting lid

Direction

- ❖ Place the half roll paper towel in the airtight container
- ❖ Get a small bowl, combine all the ingredients, mix well and pour over the paper towel. Until it is wet
- ❖ Allow to sit for a while and then remove the cardboard in the center of the paper towel
- ❖ Use as needed

DISCLAIMER: These recipes for the hand sanitizer and wipes are not to replace proper handwashing with soap rather they are meant to be handy when handwashing is not available. In addition, these homemade recipes has a general agreed natural antiviral properties, however its full efficacy has not been lab tested. As usual, consult your doctor or physician before using any home remedy on yourself or your family.